KEYS TC
RAISING CHILDREN
with
DYSLEXIA
and
ADHD

Concheta Gladmon

DEDICATION

This book is dedicated to my son, Gerard
who struggled with Adhd and Dyslexia in his early
years. Through his struggles he learned to cope
and enjoy life. I wrote this book to encourage parents
and their child to do the same. If Gerard can live life to the
fullest with success, so can your child. As his mom, I have such
admiration for him for showing me that life's challenges
could and would not conquer his spirit.

I would like to thank my Mom and family for
supporting me during my writing journey. I
finally finished and I hope that I have
made you proud. Thank you Garrison for
blessing me with a wonderful son who
touches and inspires everyone he meets.
Rest in Peace Dad.
I love you.

Table of Contents

Introduction 1

Chapter One Infancy – Toddler Years 2

Chapter Two Elementary Years 5

Occupational Therapy 5

ADHD/Dyslexia Diagnosis 7

Chapter Three Middle School 17

Chapter Four High School 27

ADHDEarly Intervention Program 29

Chapter Five The Brain in children with ADHD 33

Home Management 33

Driving 35

Medicine 36

ADHD Coaching 37

Chapter Six Parent Advice 42

Introduction

In this book, aptly titled "Keys to Successfully Raising Children With Dyslexia and ADHD", Concheta Gladmon tells us the story of how she's learned to be a good mother to her Dyslexic child, Gerard Hearst, who was also diagnosed with ADHD. She tells the beautiful story of how Gerard is growing up quite well with the two conditions and even goes as far as telling us how she's learned to manage him and to be the solid rock on which he leans.

Concheta tells us about the challenges of raising Gerard and how she previously had a hard time adjusting to the role of raising him due to her tight schedule. A schedule that forced her to multitask between studying and carrying out research for her Masters degree all the while raising a child who was different. She describes to us how despite his difference he has been able to relate well with everyone and become a darling to all those with whom he associates day in day out. Most would opine that his good nature, happy demeanor, and good manners has made him a darling among his friends and teachers and rightfully so.

The book also details to us how support and love for such a special child can go a long way in aiding their development. Concheta tells us about Gerard's awesome support system from his friends, family and teaching fraternity. Gerard happens to be a naturally impulsive person who tends to act, and then think. Read from this beautiful support diary of a book of how his support system has understood him and helped him face the world a confident young man.

As you read this book you will be educated on how best to be a parent to a specially different child and unconditionally love them. It is okay to fall but it matters only how you get up. Concheta even tells us how she fell from grace as concerns bring up and caring for her son. This book is a must read for anyone in the same shoes be it as a parent, a friend or a teacher. Added bonus, it's a good read. My desire is that you enjoy it and learn from it.

Chapter One
Infancy – Toddler Years

"Logic will get you from A to B. Imagination will take you everywhere." ~ Albert Einstein

No matter how much we try to structure our lives and be in control of everything that happens to us, events will occur that we did not anticipate or imagine and will serve as tests to our strength and character as a person. My son was born on the 8th day of the blistering hot month of July in the year 1999. The nurses pronounced him to be a healthy baby boy at 7lbs and 8ounces. He was my first child, so like every new mother I doted on his every move, crawl, coo, and smile. His father and I named him Gerard Garrison Hearst. My career had been my focus during my early twenties and I delayed pregnancy until I was well advanced in my career and in age – much to my family's chagrin. I was 28 when I gave birth to him and my family members breathed a sigh of relief when it happened. Gerard's father had been my boyfriend since the age of 16 and we were engaged at the time of his birth. We were high school and college sweethearts; however our relationship did not last. Our ideas about relationships and commitment were not aligned. We decided to part ways and still remain the best parents that we could be for our son.

Despite the rocky start to motherhood I was extremely happy to be a new mom and embraced the challenge with a huge smile on my face. Gerard slept well when I brought him home from the hospital and was a sweet baby that I enjoyed spending my day with when I was not working. I decided to stay home with him until he turned 18 months, at which time I enrolled in graduate school. I placed him in day care and his paternal grandmother would keep him during the week too. He was a joy to watch as he was all boy; running, jumping, falling, and constantly on the go. Gerard would run around with all of his cousins, ignoring all my yelling, and play well with his friends. He also napped at least two hours during the day and slept well at night.

As a toddler, Gerard was a joy to be around and watch grow. He was not a temperamental child. Even though I was a first time mother, he did not create a challenge that I could not fix or soothe which had me feeling like an award winning mother. When he was one year old, I was a personal trainer in her late twenties, so I had a great amount of energy. I placed him in the Apple Tree Academy daycare when he turned 20 months old. He really enjoyed going to school and I never noticed that he was a busy child because, well, the plan was to keep him busy throughout the day.

We took daily park trips in the neighborhood as well as daily trips downtown to feed the birds. I loved the outdoors (and since Gerard came out of me I assumed he would too), so I bought a bike and took him on adventurous trails of nature. Boy was I right about him, Gerard and I would go to the bike trail and ride for hours so that he could see nature and feel the Georgia breeze on his face. You could see from his smiles how much he loved those trips. He would often fall asleep on the way home from our bike rides. He was a playful toddler who loved Blues Clues simply because he loved to draw and write in his "handy dandy" notebook. He could hold a conversation with literally everyone that he met. He never met a stranger that he did not like or approach to speak to. People often commented to me that his personality and attitude was the nicest that they had seen since the early eighties when children were respectful. I would tell them that he was born like that; I never had to teach him to be respectful - God made him that way and I loved it. His manners were admired by me, family members, and others that he met.

As Gerard grew older, he became more active, but nothing that I could not handle. I noticed that he had a huge amount of energy when we would arrive home in the afternoon. At night he sometimes had a hard time going to sleep at his bedtime. I knew that it was important to fill his days with more activities to ensure that he was tired by nightfall so he could get the amount of sleep needed to be productive during the day. In a desperate attempt to give him more play time and wear out his energy, I registered him for the

Little Gym twice a week. He played and interacted with children his age and the instructor made sure he kept him busy. My son really loved going there on Tuesday and Thursday afternoons. The Little Gym was the key to having him tired and ready for bed. He had less energy when we arrived home; mission accomplished!

When Gerard was three he advanced to the three year old room in daycare. His teachers Ms. Amanda and Ms. Fushia adored him as he was very sweet to them and the other children in the classroom. They told me that he did not take naps during the two hour nap period but instead he would play with his shoe by tying and untying the laces. Now I had noticed his laces were always tied different than the way I tied them in the morning but I just thought that was funny, picturing him tying and untying his shoes for two hours. His teachers asked me if I could bring coloring books and crayons for him to color during nap time, so I took the crayons and coloring book to school for him to find his inner artist. Gerard may have colored only once in that book during the entire year.

His teachers never complained about him not napping though. I figure that if he remained quiet on his mat, then they were ok with him not taking naps. Happily and hopeful, Gerard graduated to Pre-K thanks to his teachers who were great with him and patient. I was so thankful that there were never any complaints from his teachers about his napping or talking. He seemed to be the teacher's pet. They also did not complain about his ability to climb and jump on objects that boys loved to jump on. These were actions that my son surely exhibited, but I could handle it considering I thought all boys were the same. I was just extremely thankful that he was not defiant, moody, or had conduct and behavioral issues like some children experience.

Chapter Two
Elementary Years

"I get bored very easily and that is a good motivator. I think everyone should have Dyslexia and ADD." ~ Paul Orfalea

Kindergarten was a big step for him. He was super excited that he was going to be on the hall with the 1st graders. I guess that really made him feel like he was older and more mature. It is well known that if a student with dyslexia can reach the age of fourteen or fifteen with a healthy sense of self-esteem and a realistic acceptance of both personal strengths and weaknesses, that student is more likely to enjoy a happy and successful life. As he entered kindergarten, he felt like he was a big kid that could finally do things on his own. During the school year the teachers suggested that he attend occupational therapy to help him focus and concentrate during the day. They noted that Gerard had a hard time paying attention and focusing in class. Occupational therapy would help him to focus and concentrate during the day.

Occupational Therapy

A few months into kindergarten, he was evaluated by the Occupational Therapist. Afterwards I met with the therapist so she could show me how to brush Gerard on his arms to help stimulate his nerves. This had to be done repeatedly throughout the day and so a routine was developed where I brushed him in the morning, the school nurse brushed him after lunch and I brushed him when he arrived home. He was also screened by a Licensed Speech Language Pathologist; he did well in semantics although he had problems with the non-literal meanings - idioms, metaphors, proverbs - and some difficulty with categories. When it came to retelling a story in sequence, phonemic awareness, following directions and recall he had a bit of a struggle. However, he was age appropriate in conversation and pragmatics.

Therapy continued over the next few weeks and the therapist gave us further instructions in stages on how to manage the condition. She asked that I encourage Gerard to hold his pencil by resting the pencil on his middle finger as this did not come naturally to him. The following week, they continued therapy and she suggested drawing and taking snips by using the ends of scissors when cutting. I was chastised for not brushing four times a day as this was a very important part of the process. I must admit that I brushed 2 times but not three times a day; it was difficult taking care of Gerard and his two year old brother while I was in school working on my Master's Degree, so I completely forgot at times. Also Gerard remained a happy playful child so I wasn't sure what the entire therapist's fuss was about. She noted that she had seen some mild changes in therapy, but cautioned that I would actually make focus and concentration and impulsivity worse if I did not brush a minimum of four times a day. I was to brush him in the morning before school, at lunchtime when he got home from school, and at dinnertime/bedtime. Brushing my son's arm four times a day was non-negotiable and I had to keep it up to see results. In addition to this, she wanted him to swing on a tire swing at home or on the playground about four to five times a week.

The volume of instructions from the occupational therapist – and she absolutely insisted on each one - caused me to begin to despair as I could not begin to imagine where I would find the time to carry out each and every one of them. To be honest, I am not sure if the occupational therapy worked. He seemed the same smart, talkative, kid that had fun wherever he visited. However, he continued with the therapy until he was promoted to first grade. He seemed to really hit his stride when he got into first grade. This was largely thanks to his teacher who did all she could to bring out the best in him. His first grade teacher adored him and would always tell me during the fall and spring parent/teacher conferences that Gerard had a good heart and personality. The hugs which she gave him every morning when he arrived at school and every afternoon when he was leaving went a long way for him and she never mentioned him being busy or needing occupational therapy.

ADHD/Dyslexia Diagnosis

Without any incident in first grade, my son was promoted to second grade. I can still vividly recall his excitement during the summer as he was about to progress to second grade. As luck would have it, his second grade teacher had a Masters in Reading which would prove highly beneficial in my son's education. During the month of October she approached me in the school hallway and asked me if I had worked on reading with my son and heard him read to which I replied that I had been working with him since he was four years old. She asked me if I noticed that he is a slow reader and I told her that it was one of the things which concerned me greatly (and which I tried not to think too much about). She said he may have dyslexia and referred me to a Psychologist who works with children who have dyslexia. I was somewhat shocked to hear that my son could have dyslexia. Although I had heard of the condition, I had never met anyone who actually had dyslexia. I looked at my carefree son who was always full and laugh and my heart constricted when I thought of him having to struggle with dyslexia. I immediately wanted to know everything about it and find out what the issues could be with him.

I called the psychologist whom his second grade teacher recommended to me and set up the earliest appointment available. She told me to let my son think that he was going to a place to play with Legos as she informed me that she would study him in such actions similar to playing with Legos. The meeting went smoothly and by the end of it she confirmed my fears. Gerard was diagnosed with dyslexia and she made recommendations on what I needed to do immediately:

1. The first suggestion was to meet with the school and determine how to help Gerard given the test results. He would need help in reading and math, so I had to explore what services the school had, or if they had services outside of the school for such cases.

2. The single most important intervention for reading would be proper instruction with methods proven to help. Gerard needed explicit teaching programs and would not benefit from implicit methods of teaching. He still needed particular help with phonetics; he had some individual reading skills mastered, but was not proficient enough to be a fluent reader, as the reading material would become more challenging.

3. Any multi-sensory programs based on Orton Gillingham methods would help him strengthen his reading skills; any other program will not be helpful nor any tutor/teacher not trained specifically in these areas. This is a true statement considering we spent a lot of money during his two years at Sylvian Learning Center but he never received the help that he needed.

4. Based on his diagnosis of specific learning disability, Gerard was eligible for extra time on both standardized and classroom exams with significant reading, writing, and/or math demands. He would also benefit from a quiet testing environment. If he ran out of time on a test, he could write, "Ran out of time" across the top of the paper and turn it in with the rest of class. Then he and his teacher could set up a time to finish the test assignment without drawing attention to him.

5. Until he had proper intervention in reading, all tests would be read to him as well as the questions on the test. This will ensure that tests are grading his knowledge and not just his reading ability.

6. Gerard was not to be graded down for spelling errors, unless he took a spelling test.

7. Books were to be made available on CD or read to him.

The psychologist also informed us about other forms of intervention which would be useful in handling ADHD:

1. There was medication for the treatment of ADHD which could have been pursued but we decided not to take that route.

2. The Test of Variable Attention (TOVA) can be given a second time on medication and the results compared with the TOVA results not on medication. Seeing as we were not going with medication, we did not pursue this either.

3. There is no medication without side effects. However, psychostimulants are proven to have no long-term side effects if taken at prescribed dosages. We also chose not to pursue this.

4. She suggested that I should use a positive reward system to assist in the completion of homework and reduce the power struggle between Gerard and I. I learned that breaking down homework into smaller, rewardable tasks that lead to the completion of homework would be more effective.

5. It was recommended that I try counseling with parents in behavior management techniques and coping ideas that would help Gerard reach his potential. Early intervention is the key to maximizing positive outcomes for him. I am a strong person so I decided that I could handle any behavioral issues.

6. We decided to keep extra textbooks at home in order to provide more ready access to materials both at home and at school.

7. I was to have him work only on one task at a time or a step larger at a time. This action helped with greater organization and planning.

8. I had to say his name and ensure that I had eye contact before I started t to talk to him. I was to speak slowly, fully enunciating each word in order for him to understand. Gerard was not to be given multiple tasks at one time – no more than two things at a time. I had to keep my words direct and watch what I said so that I did not go off on a tangent explaining things as that would have him confused.

9. It was very important to look for positives. I would need to provide immediate feedback to him each time he accomplished the desired behavior or achievement, no matter how small the accomplishment.

10. It was extremely important to praise Gerard in public, and reserve all reprimands for private.

11. I needed to learn the characteristics of ADHD, especially inconsistent performance, and accept those as real cognitive deficits. I also learned to not attribute poor performance to laziness, poor motivation, or internal traits.

With the test results, I was reassured about the few times that I worked with him during the summer and thought he was reading a bit slower than expected. I can remember one incident working with him when he was in Kindergarten. I bought the book "How to Teach Your Child to Read in 100 Days". Gerard and I worked for 30 minutes every day during the summer. He was eager to read and ready learn every day. He and I would sit side by side on the couch while my 1 year old took a nap. He learned quickly and picked up on the new letters and words that were introduced. Soon he was reading paragraphs and passages like a pro, a lot of high fives were shared as we progressed. We bonded through daily reading since we sat on the couch, turned off the T.V. and had only the sounds of his and my voice resonating throughout the house. I encouraged him during the process and at the end of August he finished the book.

I decided to move fast after the diagnosis of dyslexia and ADHD. As I mentioned earlier, his second grade teacher had a Master's Degree in Reading, so she was able to help him if he had issues with reading and comprehension. She and I scheduled a meeting to talk about the best way that we could collaborate to give him the support that he would need to be successful. She offered to provide him with one on one sessions that would help him understand the lesson for the day. I followed the advice of the psychologist and registered him for the multi-sensory dyslexia facility which used the Orton-Gillingham method developed by Samuel Orton and Anna Gillingham in the 1930's. It involves a multisensory approach which was very useful for teaching children with ADHD. The approach helps students develop the ability to break down the written code of language. It is often delivered as one on one tutoring or in small group instruction.He attended the facility twice a week for an hour and immediately warmed up to the instructors (like he always did) who worked to teach him the multisensory way of learning, making it easier for him to grasp what he was being taught.

Soon it was time for him to begin third grade. In his third grade year, I had a meeting with the administrators. Third grade was not the most successful year for Gerard as he was required to learn and absorb much more than he was used to and this was very challenging for him. He had a wonderful teacher who was extremely patient and kind. Gerard also had classmates that he had been in school with since Kindergarten, so he felt comfortable in school. However, he complained throughout the school year that he felt stupid and dumb. His self-esteem was extremely low and I had to put extra effort into praising him in all efforts so that he knew he was loved and valued. I would look him in the eyes and tell him that he was neither dumb nor stupid but rather he was intelligent and smart.

My efforts seemed futile however as I don't think he believed that because he would still reiterate his thought to me weekly. He had problems with reading and had to go back over the reading material several times and this made him to dread having to read aloud, so I informed the teacher that he was not comfortable with reading in front of the class. She was very understanding and agreed not to ask him to read aloud. This went a long way to boosting his self-esteem and become his former cheerful self.

Second grade Math was also very hard for Gerard as the work was word problems and there was a lot of reading involved. I think organizing the information in the word problems and following the sequence of steps to find the answer was the hardest part for him. My heart began to ache for him because I knew how hard he was trying to learn. I made the decision not to tell him that he had dyslexia because I felt he was too young and would not understand. Instead I tried to explain to him that his brain was wired a bit differently from other students and it may take him longer to learn, but he would get it in the end. In math he seemed to have trouble reading the test material and organizing the information. He also had problems writing down answers; therefore, timed tests were hard for him to finish.

I told him the famous story of the Tortoise and the Hare to illustrate to him that the people who are determined don't have to be the fastest as long as they keep going to the finish line.I explained to him that it doesn't matter if other children finish tests or assignments before him; the important thing was for him to keep focus and finish on his own time without worrying about others. I explained to him that some students may finish early because they may not have studied and perhaps they could be writing anything just to finish the test. He understood what I was saying and that put a smile on his face and I could see that he was inspired by the story. He promised me that he would only focus on his test or assignment and try as hard as he could to always pass. That's all I wanted to hear. He was very smart then, but I get it; he felt that he was not normal. He felt like he was in the room full of normal students and he was not understanding the lesson or concept that was taught. He wondered why his classmates understood what was taught and he could not comprehend it at all.

Every day I made sure to reaffirm to him that he was extremely smart. I wanted to keep grinding that into his head so that he could eventually repeat it over and over to himself. I wanted to help him develop a positive self-image and self-esteem; I had him focus on his strengths, such as football. He liked the praise that he received in football and track, which in turn helped him develop self-confidence in school. As I mentioned, my son loves to draw. His artwork is incredible considering the art is totally unique and one of a kind. He loves showing his work to family and friends and I could see how much of a sense of pride this filled him with.

During the cold winter month of March, I had another meeting with the administrators which included my son's teacher this time around. They informed me that they did not have the resources to help him in fifth grade so I would have to look into public school since it offered all the resources that would help him in school. I could not understand why a private school did not have the necessary resources that would help my son, but I did not complain because this move would save me money. I dreaded explaining to my son that he would have to leave the school he had attended for many years and leave the many faces that he had seen for all of those years. Surprisingly, he was ok with leaving and moving to public school. In fact he was very excited at the prospect of riding the big yellow school bus along with the other students. We live in the suburb of Atlanta where the public schools have well trained administration and teachers. I knew that he would be in good hands when I sent him off in August.

I called his new school early in August to schedule a meeting with the counselor and administration that would handle the 504 meeting. Gerard is protected by the Individuals with Disabilities Education Act, Section 504 of the Rehabilitation Act, and American with Disabilities Act. IDEA provides federal funding to public schools to support a "free and appropriate education" (FAPE) to students. Section 504 applies to any person who has a physical or mental impairment which substantiality limits one or more major activities. The major activity is defined as "learning" and "reading". I also learned that Section 504 protects people with disabilities from discrimination in private or public programs that receive federal funds. Section 504 requires that Gerard is educated in the "least restrictive environment" (LRE). This means he is educated with his peers who do not have disabilities. Once the school knew my son had dyslexia, they were legally obligated to provide him with services and accommodations at no cost. This was good news to hear. To receive accommodations in public school dyslexia falls into the category of special learning disability as introduced in the Individuals with Disabilities Education Act (IDEA).

The meeting consisted of the Assistant Principal, Counselor, and Student Support Teacher (SST). This was all new to me considering my son had been in private school his entire life from Kindergarten. I was not nervous or jittery as I was fully prepared. I had all of my paperwork from the previous testing. I brought along the psychoeducational test which had everything that they would need to place him in the class with a teacher who was knowledgeable about ADHD and dyslexia.I knew that I was representing as the executive parent; I had self confidence that I was ultimately in charge of the meeting what would help provide proper education for Gerard.

I am the case manager of my son's life and must be a proactive parent prepared to take charge. I knew that they would have a lot of questions about him therefore Iwent for that meeting prepared to field each and every one of those questions to their satisfaction. They asked questions about his behavior and temperament and I answered that he was extremely sweet and eager to please any person. I told them that he loves to meet people and make friends fast because he is under the impression that everyone is his friend. They read the information that the Psychologist provided that described him and they stated that "they couldn't wait to meet him". I left the meeting feeling accomplished that I had placed him in a school that would not only teach him, but work with him one on one to help him become successful.

After the meeting, we had three more weeks before school started. We traveled to the beach for one week, then came back and started football practice for the next two weeks. Fourth grade here we come. My son started fourth grade excited, ready to meet new friends and teachers. To my happiness, he had a male teacher who was extremely patient and nice. Soon he had a few friends that he came home talking about every day. In early September, I received a letter in the mail reading he would start Math and Language Arts Early Intervention Program (EIP) in October. Throughout September he continued making new friends and learning in fourth grade.

October rolled around and he began EIP where he was in both classes with eight students. After he started taking the EIP classes he was finally able to comprehend math well enough to explain it to me when asked. He also understood what was happening in language artsandI was thrilled that he was receiving the help that he needed to succeed. Gerard continued going to the multi-syllables facility twice a week the entire year. He was making progress and beginning to feel confident. Fourth grade was a blast for him. I never once received any complaints from him about feeling dumb or stupid. I volunteered to come to his class a few times and had a chance to get to know the students. He was in a great class with lovely and fun classmates. They even had a pet hamster named snickers that we took home twice from Friday afternoon to Monday morning. He continued EIP every day of the week until the beginning of May. Gerard never had an issue and felt successful at all times.

In what seemed like a blink of an eye, the summer of fourth grade was upon us and it felt good to know that he was confident about himself and learning. As was our custom, we spent the summer together as a family going on several fun adventures such as travelling, running track and fishing. When August began, I scheduled the requisite meeting with administrators to complete his 504 form and accommodations. As a mom, I was relieved that I could provide the help that he needed to feel successful in school. I was actually really proud of myself because some people may feel anxious to meet with administrators or teachers, but I was not afraid considering my son needed help in school and I was well equipped and knowledgeable about his condition. When school started I learned that he had an older female teacher who loved to read and had a Masters in Reading and I was delighted because I knew that she would be doubly perfect. I felt she was perfect because she was older and could work one on one with him when he read in order to comprehend the subject. My mom told me years ago that older teachers have more patience because they've been teaching for a longer period of time. As it turned out, my mom was right (she usually is). She was friendly and very approachable during the 504 meeting and also throughout the school year.

Gerard was looking forward to fifth grade simply because the students rotated classes. He could now go next door to Science class and down the hall to Math. He also liked the fifth grade class as there were about five football players and one track runner. He felt comfortable around kids that were sports oriented as he could identify with them more easily and he was not slower than they were when it came to comprehending sports. Due to his scores on the CRCT, Gerard was placed in EIP Math and Language Arts. He had very good grades in both classes as the small group sessions were working. Again, he felt very confident and successful in school. To my happiness, he was promoted to sixth grade without difficulty.

Chapter Three
Middle School

"Don't chase people, be yourself, do your own thing and work hard. The right people - the right ones who really belong in your life - will come to you and stay." ~ Will Smith

We went on vacation that summer as usual. Gerard made it to Junior Olympics in the 100 meter dash, so he was headed to Detroit, Michigan in July. After Junior Olympics, he started football practice for the sixth grade feeder team. As always, he was excited and ready to play football and see his friends, but not excited for school itself. Like all children, he did not want summer to end. I set a meeting for mid-August to discuss the 504 form. Administrators gave him all accommodations that ranged from more time on assignments and tests to a quiet area to take a test. The only thing that I did not know or expect was that the EIP program did not extend into middle school. However, a small group had been created in Middle School for students with a 504 form.

Gerard tested well on the CRCT, so well that he tested out of Language Arts small group. He was not happy about this testing news. He asked me if I could talk to the counselor to place him back in the small group because he felt that he would have to work harder. I told him I would not talk to a counselor and he would stay in the class because the CRCT provided proof that he was capable of doing well and passing the course. He was not too thrilled with my decision. This is just the news that I wanted to read. His Psychologist told us if we kept him attending the multi-syllables facility for two years and place him in small group for two years that he would be able to mainstream into regular classes. I was smiling ear to ear, but he wasn't cracking a smile because he wanted it easy. I told him that I knew his potential and he knew he was extremely smart. I did not fall for the "but mom you know I'm dumb and stupid" trick. He would receive small group help in only Math. Gerard's test scores were average, but luckily the school felt that he still needed help in math.

I decided to tell Gerard that he had dyslexia in sixth grade. I felt that he was now mature enough to handle the condition and could understand how having dyslexia would affect his life. He not only knew that his brain was wired differently; he also now knew he was diagnosed with dyslexia. I also explained him that ADHD was something that made a person different, but that differences are good and the difference of ADHD is a gift. I told him that because he is different from other children this may sometimes make life harder for him. I tried to make him understand that he had traits that made him really good at some things, and his differences would one day serve the world in important, needed ways. I needed him to see that these disabilities did not make him less of a person or reduce his potentials to become someone great and influential in society.

Studies show that there is no agreement among experts as to what constitutes dyslexia. What I know for sure is dyslexia is a genetic, brain-based characteristic that results in difficulty connecting the sounds of spoken language to written words. The word dyslexia is derived from the Greek words *dys* which refers to a difficulty, and *lexia*, which refers to a use of words. The condition called dyslexia refers to a difficulty using words or language, and people with this condition are called dyslexics. The core of dyslexic's issues is the difficulty with phonological awareness, which is the ability to appreciate that spoken language, is made up of individually distinct sound units. Dyslexia causes problems for people in using oral or written language. These problems may occur in reading, writing, spelling, math, speaking, and listening. Children who have dyslexia are often mistakenly thought of as lazy, stupid, or dumb. The truth is that dyslexics are usually bright and creative. In fact Most of them have average or above average intelligence.Those who have dyslexia can be highly independent. Dyslexia is also characterized by a set of strengths in one or more of the following areas: verbal, social, spatial, narrative, kinesthetic, visual, mathematical, or musical skills. As I mentioned previously, Gerard's strengths are verbal, social, kinesthetic, and visual

Gerard's Symptoms

People who have dyslexia have a lack of awareness of phonemes in written or spoken language. Phonemes are the smallest units of language. For example, the "b" in book is a phoneme. Considering they lack phonological awareness, dyslexics tend to have trouble connecting letters with their correct sounds, distinguishing whether sounds are the same or different, separating words into their parts, and blending parts of words. Educators consider these types of symptoms of dyslexia. Confusing letters or words; when reading or writing my Gerard might mistake "duck" for "buck", for example. When doing math computation, he might mistake"25" for "52". He would also mistake words for similar words, such as "met" for "wet". In math, he might mistake "9" for "6".

Dyslexics have problems with spelling; Gerard constantly erases, crosses out and writes over misspelled words. From what I understand this problem is because he has trouble connecting letters with sounds and distinguishing the separate sounds in words. For example when writing "pack", he may misspell it as "back". He also has problems with sequencing in the sense that his letters are likely to be different sizes and tend to be reversed or written over. One thing that I find funny; he writes on the back of a piece of paper and always think it's the front side. I remind him of this every time he writes, but he smiles as continues to write.

Gerard also has difficulty following instructions; he has problems remembering completing chores, and school assignments. There are times that I ask him to clean his bathroom and make his bed. Hours later when I check his room, nothing is done and when I turn to him blazing hot with fury he would simply tell me that he forgot and I could see in his eyes that it was the truth. Gerard definitely has problems with organization. His room is normally a mess if I don't have time to clean it. He leaves his dirty clothes on the floor forgetting to place them in the hamper, he does not put his shoes in his closet and he definitely does not do any form of folding, arrangement or hanging of clean clothes. This makes organizing his room and bathroom a veritable uphill task.

Luckily I run a professional organization company in Atlanta; so putting items in their proper place is what I do for a living. One thing that I found helpful is that I started listing his household chores and assignments and texting it to his iPhone so that he can put it in his calendar. I tell him all the time that I feel sorry for his roommate whenever he attends college. I hope Gerard's roommate is cleaner than him. Since my son has difficulty with the concept of time passing, he struggles to get to school on time and often forgets his backpack and binder. After noticing his lack of organization and time-management, I developed a way to help him become successful at school and home.

Strategies for Success

Before Gerard heads to bed, he has his brother help him pack his backpack for the next day. Planners and IPhone reminders are a helpful tool for keeping track of important dates of assignments. Tape reading material was helpful for him considering he does not like reading.Helistened to a tape while following along in his books. He could rewind the tapes and go back to review any parts that confused him. I also encouraged Gerard to make use of his Section 504 and ask the teacher to allow for more time on tests, assignments, class work, and projects. He also benefited when his teachers read his test aloud so that he could look at the words of the questions while hearing them spoken.

The computer is Gerard's best friend. I have learned that dyslexic students improve their communication skills drastically when they begin to use computers to compensate for their dyslexia-based difficulties in diverse and creative ways. Several functions available on computer software which most people take for granted are lifelines to Gerard and people with hearing and sight disabilities when it comes to communicating in writing: auto text, spell check, voice recognition, creating text, use of the keyboard, word prediction and reading out text, just to mention a few. Computers have been invaluable for offering varied ways for Gerard to get his thoughts down on paper and to be creative with his writing, with graphics, canned-in-pictures, time lines, and animation.

Computers also helped Gerard with organization as it offered the possibility of keeping weekly, monthly, and semester calendars on the screen. Conversely, computers can do the reading, scan books and read them aloud while the person follows along with the words on the screen. Note, there isn't one particular computer application created for dyslexics which can be used generally because people will feel the effects of dyslexia in different ways. So it is more of taking advantage of the functions and adaptations provided by the computer in order to make reading and writing easier for them. Tips to help: double spacing text, using the voice recognition system built into the system, changing the screen background and contrast settings. Many dyslexic people are sensitive to the glare of the usual white background on a page, white board or computer screen, making text bigger and using a bolder color are some of the ways computers can be helpful to someone who is dyslexic. Dyslexics can use text-to-speech programs to proof read, reduce visual stress and increase the accuracy of their work.

Dyslexic students usually struggle to get their thoughts into writing on the page. They may have wonderful ideas and topics to write in but are not able to write them down. I suggest making use of voice recognition software to combat this problem. If used the right way, they will find that they can speak at the same speed at which you type – sometimes faster. The text to speech function is also available for them to have the text they write down read back to them. This takes away the pressure of how to put down ideas and allows them to focus their energies on coming up with great ideas while the computer takes care of the rest. So the ideas are read out to the computer using voice recognition, and then what has been typed on the screen is read aloud to you using text to speech to crosscheck and make sure that the computer got down the right things. This saves the dyslexic a whole lot of time and energy and builds confidence that they can communicate effectively.

One of the most valuable systems for dyslexics is books on tape. The richest source of books on tapes is Reading for the Blind and Dyslexic of which my son is a member. The organization has over seventy-five thousand recorded volumes including many textbooks in just about all subjects, plus fiction, drama, and poetry.

Gerard did not really understand how his brain could be so different compared to his classmates and friends. One day we drove to the neighborhood library to pick up a book "What is Dyslexia", which is a book Explaining Dyslexia for Kids and Adults to Use Together by Alan M. Hultquist. This explained dyslexia to Gerard in the ways that he would be able to understand about his body. I felt relief that he was finally able to understand that he was not born stupid or dumb; he had a genetic disorder which he could not wash or wish away. He asked me why I didn't tell him earlier. I told him that I felt he would not understand the disorder and he would be overly dramatic at times and after a few seconds during which I imagine he was trying to decide whether to forgive me or accuse me of ruining his life he said, "Yeah, you are right" and I was able to breathe easy. It was very encouraging to him to learn that Albert Einstein had dyslexia because Einstein is one of his favorite scientists.

With happiness and glee, sixth grade was a great year. Gerard was placed in a small group for Math. During mid-year he did not score well on a math assessment, so his counselor asked me if I could begin bringing him to school early for a thirty minute help session. The session was scheduled for Mondays, Wednesdays, and Thursdays and to say the least, Gerard was not thrilled to hear this. He was not happy that he would have to wake up early and go to school early either. Although he did not enjoy going to the sessions, I felt good that he understood the math concepts and his grade increased. He was a trooper and wanted to be successful and attended help sessions with a smile.

During the summer I received a letter stating Gerard's test scores for math did not require that he attend small group anymore. As you can guess, he was not happy to read that information. I commended him for testing well. He was not happy considering he felt that he would have to work harder in class. I reassured him that he would still receive help from his teacher because he would have the 504 that stated he had dyslexia and accommodations. Like usual, he wanted me to contact the counselor and ask her to place him back in small group math but I told him that was not going to happen because I knew that he was smart enough and could now do the work without the help of the small group classes. He got really upset and replied thathe should have just marked anything on the test so that he could get back into small group. I told him that the test showed that he was smart and capable of performing in class and being successful in school. Seventh and eighth grade went by really fast like lightning. I met with administrators and we agreed upon the Section 504and they provided Gerard with the same accommodations as in previous years. He was promoted to ninth grade. High school here we come!

Identifying Strengths

During the process of learning Gerard had dyslexia and while helping him stay organized for school I was able to assess his strengths and attributes that would help make him successful. I allowed him to embrace his core skills which included visual, kinesthetic, and social skills. Since he is a visual learner, he enrolled in art class; socially, he is friendly to everyone, and kinesthetics wise, he plays football, runs track and wrestles. I made sure to emphasize his strengths every day as well as praise him for a job well done whenever he used his skills.

There is no child that is born without gifts. Children who are diagnosed with having attention deficit disorder are no exception to this rule. However, their gifts and talents may be hidden under all that energy and will require patience to identify and even more work to let lose. Parents can be overwhelmed when they learn this and they may not know how to go about bringing out the best in that child. First and foremost you must determine to commit to showing your child constant love and affection. Doing this requires time as you will have to interact with your child and watch and listen to him.

The goal is to capture the essence and spirit of your child as you spend quality and quantity time with him in order to get to know who he really is and what he possesses. Before the world begins to label your child based on her actions it is important for you to have the knowledge of who your child actually is. By the time your child starts kindergarten he will be classified as friendly or withdrawn, engaging or taciturn, klutzy or athletic, stupid or smart. Psychologists and therapists will generalize and simplify and lump your child into a category based on his symptoms, and this is their job. It is up to you, however, to hold on to what you know in your heart about your child and remind him of this every step of the way.

Even 'normal' kids can grow up disconnected from their families. The presence of material things in a home does not fill in the hole created by a lack of emotional connection to other members of the family. A child who is connected feels like a part of something bigger than himself, he feels safe and secure in the cocoon of love spun by his parents and caregivers. This connection is even more important for children with ADHD as it helps them transition more smoothly into society when the time comes. Building this connection requires spending time with your child as I mentioned earlier. During this time you are not to be focused on giving direct orders or trying to get them to do one thing or the other. You are to just be there for them, watch him, and listen to him. Get to know him as he also gets to know you and know you are there for him and that he can always depend on you. It is vital for him to know that you are in his corner no matter what the rest of the world may be saying or how they may be treating him.

Gerard is a wonderful person. I am super proud to be his mom. He brings excitement and energy to his brother and me and he has the ability to look at things with a fresh perspective.I ask my son to dream big at all times and to work hard to make that dream a reality. I know with all of my heart that he will excel at all things even if he may fall a bit; simply because he gives 100% at all times in life. I help him by setting educational goals, such as registering him for art class since he draws in his spare time and even when he is at school. He feels his strengths are in athletics, so we allow him to play football to achieve his dream of going to college on a football scholarship. He understands that his other strength is speed, so he runs track because he is aware that college coaches seek running backs that are fast. His school accommodates him well which showcases his strengths; therefore allowing him to succeed. I tell him all the time that his dreams should be as bold and powerful as his classmates.

Certain factors have been listed by dyslexics as personal and emotional success. These factors include tenacity, confidence, positive self-image, a realistic acceptance of the personal struggles and shortcomings associated with dyslexic learning challenges, but also a deliberate focusing on personal strengths and areas of special interest, supportive home and school environments and a supportive network of friends. These factors fall into the internal and external supports. Confidence and self-worth develops when dyslexics learn to recognize and use their strengths. Gerard found that knowing his strengths developed confidence in him during his years of academic struggle because it made him feel useful and valuable.

Dyslexics are a small 10% of people, 35% entrepreneurs, and 41% of prisoners. I was surprised and also intrigued to read these numbers. I am my son's advocate and encourager, so he will not be that person in prison sitting and waiting on a release date. There are several key traits among dyslexic entrepreneurs. The first is a remarkable sense of vision for their business. They have a clear idea of where they are going and what they are doing. Second is a confident and persistent attitude. Third is the ability to ask for and engage the help of others. They have no problem surrounding themselves with people who are good at their jobs. The fourth trait is excellent oral communication, which they use to inspire staffs. What they lack in written communication, they more than make up for in speech. The employees are energized by them. A fifth and final strength trait is that many successful dyslexic entrepreneurs use their intuition a lot.

Every year I build a relationship with my son's teachers, counselors, and administrators. I want them as my allies so that we can help my son accomplish his goals in school. I have always had great communication with my son's teachers and counselors. They email or call me whenever he is missing an assignment or even when he seems distracted in class. We work as a unit to get him back on track. He is allowed five days to turn in any late assignments without there being a deduction in his grade. He can also write at the top of any paper given to him by teachers that he "needs more time". I want teachers to know that I am doing my job at home to help my son in any way possible.

Chapter Four
High School

"If my mind can conceive it and my heart can believe it - then I can achieve it." ~ Muhammad Ali

The period from mid adolescence to young adulthood is a critical time for individuals with dyslexia. During these years they must become increasingly responsible for their own organization, learning, and significance in life and school. Students with dyslexia must first and foremost develop the ability to identify and use their ideal learning style. Gerard is a kinesthetic, visual, and tactile learner. Staying organized and using time efficiently are also key components to achieving success in high school; examples include reminders on their cell phone and planners.

Without any obstacles, Gerard made it to high school. I think I was more scared for him than he was to be in high school around older kids. He had no problems blending in with his classmates and older students. I think playing sports helped him transition well considering majority of the kids at his school were athletic and participated in dual sports. I met with administrators and his new counselor in August. They looked at his file and we discussed his condition and the accommodations needed. Since they did not know him, they wanted to know about his behavior and medicine. I explained that he had no behavioral issues and did not take medicine for ADHD. He was granted the same accommodations that he has had since 4th grade. When school work started I noticed that he struggled in ninth grade Language Arts and Math. I communicated with his teachers to let them know my concerns about his grades. Remember we were allies for his success, so they offered to have him come to school early to attend their help sessions. Gerard knew he needed to attend those sessions, so I did not have a problem convincing him to wake up early to show up. As time went on his grades improved with the help of his teachers. I also had him review his work at home to make it fresh in his brain. Ninth grade was a successful year for him at school, in sports, and at home.

Whoa, now Gerard is moving to 10th grade. Boy where did the time go? As always, I met with administration, teachers, and counselor for my son's Section 504. In this meeting, the Assistant Principal focused on Gerard's ADHD. He mentioned that the previous teachers noted in the files that he was sometimes overstimulated, more so after lunch when he had a lot of energy. I admitted that I knew exactly what they were referring to because he can "spazz" when he is not busy and he usually has more energy after he eats lunch. The fact that he was also in this class with majority of his football team was a contributing factor. "Spazz" refers to a period when he becomes impulsive and talks fast and way too much. I encounter this when I pick him up from football practice. When he enters the car, he still has a lot of energy and he is ready to talk about the day. The Assistant Principal wanted to include ADHD in the Section 504. He wanted to accommodate Gerard's ADHD by offering extra time for him to complete work. He would also be allowed to stand up and go to the back of the classroom if he felt overstimulated in class. I was happy that he would receive the accommodations for ADHD and dyslexia. I was also glad that his teachers would understand his condition if he became overly busy or talkative in class.

His Psychoeducational test stated that he has ADHD with a combination of concentration/hyperactive impulsivity and was also lacking the ability to focus. He is non-problematic and has no behavioral issues. So it seems Gerard and I have survived pre-school, middle school, pre-teen and now he is in his mid-teenage years. I guess while raising him and continuing with life, the time sort of maximized on us. He is now driving and managing to cope more with his dyslexia and ADHD. He has learned social skills and better forms of social behavior. I am proud today as I watch him knowing that he will make a smooth transition into adulthood, being aware that I did everything I could to make this possible for him.

ADHDEarly Intervention Program

Attention Deficit Hyperactive Disorder (ADHD) is a condition that affects both children and adults and is characterized by problems with attention, impulsivity, and hyperactivity. ADHD cannot be cured; instead treatment focuses on managing the symptoms. I make chores more rewarding and appealing. If he wants to drive to his favorite store; I tell him that his room must be clean in order for him to drive. He does this with no problem because he will be rewarded with a drive.

ADHD has three subtypes:

1. People with inattentive type often have difficulty paying attention to detail; finishing tasks, and are easily distracted or forgetful. Inattentive ADHD involves poor concentration, where they have difficulty concentrating on things they have to look at but rather prefer listening to it. Gerard is an auditory learner who learns better when he hears information and then he can visualize it more clearly.

2. Those who have hyperactive impulsive type of ADHD, fidget and talk a lot more excessively or feel restless most of the time. They interrupt others or speak at inappropriate times, and have difficulty waiting their turn. Gerard interrupts his friend's conversation and even me when I am talking to friends. I have to remind him that he should only speak when spoken to.

3. People with combined type have a combination of inattentive and hyperactive-impulsive symptoms which culminate insocial clumsiness and learning difficulties. The approach I have found to be most successful in dealing with ADHD is to maximize Gerard's natural strengths and gifts while helping them to compensate for and cope with their weaknesses. In some ADHD children, the child is largely the impulsive type or another child can be the inattentive type, but the approach of parenting the ADHD child remains the same. The approach is to find their individual strengths and develop and encourage those strengths while providing support to help them with their challenges.

Social Clumsiness occurs when ADHD children have trouble reading social situations; they are socially 'tone deaf'. The child with ADHDappears to have an immaturity in the part of the brain responsible for social cognition and so is less able to learn socially appropriate behavior. The people who are most likely to notice are the child's contemporaries, and as a result, his peers often reject him. My son acts younger than others in his class, even though he is one of the oldest. His classmates have always called him immature. He still watches cartoon, sits in his room and draws, likes family time, is sweet to his younger brother and loves to visit grandparents. He has a few true friends in school that he can always depend on who knows him well and can tell him that he talks to much.

Identifying and knowing Gerard's strengths does not mean that I am blind to his shortcomings; as a matter of fact I make sure that he is fully aware of them and tackles them head-on. Gerard's deficits are: over-talkativeness, lack of judgment, and misinterpreting feedback. As I mentioned previously, my son's teachers and I also agree the he is overly-talkative. In class and at home, he will tone it down when asked to stop talking. In regards to lack of judgment, he talks to strangers on the street. I will ask if he knows the person that he was talking to and he will say no they just look nice and friendly. He waves and greets people when we are in the grocery store and his feelings are very hurt if that person does not respond to him.

I normally tell him that some people are not friendly and do not want to say hello. Yes, he is an extremely nice young man who has received kind words from many people. They tell me that the days when children act like him and are generous and kind are long gone. I have had people give him money as a tip when he returns their cart to the cart center or when he holds the door for them. He refuses to take the money from them. He says, he is just being himself and nice. Truly I thank God that he is the nicest boy that I know. He does not have a mean or evil part in his body.

Gerard is also not able to decipher facial expressions and body language; for example when a person is mad at him or has had enough of his jokes. I normally have to tell him that I do not want to watch anymore of his cartoon videos on YouTube simply because I have seen them at least 15 times. His youngest brother should win the 'best brother award'; he is an absolute angel with Gerard. He will sit with Gerard and watch the same video that I have watched at least 15 times without once uttering a single word of complaint.He just laughs at the video as if he has never seen it before. Gerard is one of a kind and I have definitely grown in maturity, patience, and the ability to stay calm when things seem a bit chaotic.

I was never a multi-tasker and now I pride myself on the ability to handle almost anything that he is doing or saying. At times he may throw a major curveball at me and then I become perturbed and say words that I should not say, sorry Mom and Dad. I say this to remind you that even though I am an ADHD and Dyslexic Coach, I sometimes have a hard time keeping calm when my son is in his impulsive phase. He sometimes acts before he thinks and that is sure to get him those dirty looks from me that he does not like. As an ADHD coach/consultant I am aware that his impulsivity is not under his complete control, but as a mom I feel there are certain things that he can control and he should think before he acts.However I truly know that 100% control is impossible.

With reference to the above list, Gerard has inattentive ADHD; this means that he has difficulty paying attention to detail. He is extremely quick to miss the details that are presented to him and he has to ask a few times before he can understand what is asked of him. He also has trouble finishing tasks. If I ask him to clean his room, he may begin to do it, but then he'll get sidetracked and start playing Xbox. He can get easily distracted and forgetful. There are many times when I ask him to do his household chores; he will start the chores then and a few minutes later I will check on his progress. Normally one out of five things has been completed. When

I ask what happened, he usually replies that he forgot what he was supposed to be doing at the time.

Children with impulsive ways do not do so because they are ignorant. They normally know what they should and should not do. However they respond in reflexive ways to the things that happen around them. Impulsivity happens the moment that he has to sit for some time like church. Gerard's hyperactive impulsive symptoms are noticeable when he is in a place for a while. One day, we were sitting beside one another in church and I noticed his leg was pulsating or shaking up and down. I asked him if he was nervous and he said 'no'. He had not even noticed that his leg was shaking until I pointed it out to him; he was merely trying to focus on what the pastor was saying. As I mentioned earlier, the Assistant Principal of his high school said his teachers mentioned that he talks a lot after lunch and is restless. Lunch can normally tire people and make them feel like taking a short nap, but Gerard chooses to play football with his friends after lunch, so when he enters the teacher's classroom he is still pumped and energized from football.

It is not uncommon for children with impulsivity ADHD to have broken a number of bones during their childhood. For example, Gerard has had stitches in his head because he was playing football in the house with cousins and accidentally hit his head on the kitchen table. When he talks, he gets really close to my personal space. He also touches me and others a lot and sits extremely close to us when he wants to have a conversation. Since I'm his mother the closeness and touching does not bother me, but I am sure other people may have an issue with it. I have learned that children with ADHD often cannot stop themselves from touching things or people. This need to touch people even when it is not socially acceptable stems from the fact that they are seeking input from their environment in order to better communicate their thoughts and also to understand what is being communicated to them.

Chapter Five
The Brain in children with ADHD

"I get extra time to take the test because of my ADD. Everybody's brains work differently and I just need longer for things to register."
~ Mary-Kate Olsen

One great skill that I learned from Gerard's Psychologist which helped me tremendously was the importance of getting his attention before giving him instructions. She encouraged us not to shout instructions or orders from room to room. It was imperative that I called his name and establish eye contact then give the instruction. Gerard needs me to give him one task at a time. To be honestev en though he is 16; he still requires one idea or task at a time. There is no way that I can't ask him to clean his room, pick up his socks and make his bed. I have to use clear sentences when speaking to him. Even though this task consists of everything being done in his room, it is impossible for him to remember to do all of those at the same time. I also have to make sure I use short sentences; for example, please feed the fish. Now, since that is short, sweet, and easy; the fish may get fed that day.

Home Management

It is true that children with ADHD are very challenging to raise. No parent of a child with ADHD will be able to respond to every difficulty that arises in a textbook manner. Children with ADHD often bring out the worst in their parents. Even the most patient and understanding parent is likely to make many mistakes. All that a parent of a child with ADHD should hope to achieve is to be a 'good enough' parent –a parent who tries to do his or her best, who learns from his or her mistakes, and who provides support for the child through all the difficulties that life presents.

When managing Gerard's ADHD I chose to explain to him that he had ADHD when he was in sixth grade due to his maturity level. I knew that he would not be able to understand how ADHD affected his life daily. I explained to him that different people are talented in different ways. I made sure to mention his many talents; track, wrestling, personality, football, art, and creativity. I also explained to him that I know some things are more difficult for him to do, even when he tried very hard, simply because part of his brain takes a longer time to switch on compared to other children. I explained to Gerard that I understood that he may find things difficult, but he is truly capable of doing those things. I also found the need to tell him that he would at times find it difficult to sustain his attention, control his impulsivity, and manage to win friends.

When looking at ways to help Gerard, the Psychologist told me that it is essential to look at my own needs and concerns. She reminded me that I would need help in coping with my own feelings. Luckily for my family, we had teachers, family members, and doctors who understood our concerns and my son's ADHD and dyslexia issues. I was never stressed when trying to explain Gerard's ADHD because everyone I encountered was very helpful. I took one day and one step at a time, when he was younger; I set realistic goals and concentrated on them. I concentrated on having consistent communication with his teachers and counselors. I also focused on having him feel like he could successfully perform similarly or better with his peers in school.

Children with ADHD can cause parents lots of stress. My way of reducing stress is exercise. I love to work out by jogging, participating in boot camps, and lifting weights. When I exercise endorphins take over my mind and body. I feel relieved of any tension or stress that I have in my life. I can recharge and therefore think of the positive perspective that Gerard has brought in to my life. He is such a nice and kind boy and I am happy that he is who he is because he has humbled my thoughts and changed the way that I feel about life. He brings happiness to the house and everyone that he meets.

I would definitely encourage all parents to praise your child even when it seems as if it will not change the circumstances. When Gerard said that he felt dumb and stupid; I immediately started to praise him and his efforts in school and at home. I wanted him to know that I saw the effort that he was striving for in class and at home to try to feel normal. As soon as Gerard was diagnosed with ADHD I began working with him at home. After school in the afternoon, we would sit at a table and start on his homework. I usually waited until he was finished with his afternoon snack and had at least thirty minutes to unwind before we began. I knew he needed complete quiet, so I would always work with the TV off and made sure his youngest brother was not in the room. I would revisit the topic that was previously discussed so that he would let me know if he understood the subject and we could move forward or remain on the topic. We would take breaks to let him burn off any excess energy that he had before we started work.

When working with Gerard at home, I had to make sure his team was communicating for his benefit. Gerard's team consisted of his counselor, teachers, administration, and me. I felt very comfortable in working with the Assistant Principal as he was a specialist with the 504 Section Form and accommodations. He knew and provided every accommodation that would help Gerard in school. Here is a list of effective teaching strategies that was taught to Gerard. First and foremost the teacher should have an understanding of what it is like to be a child with ADHD. Gerard's teachers understood his weaknesses and strength; therefore, they strategized and provided work to help him overcome his weaknesses.His teachers created a proper learning environment for Gerard to feel comfortable to be himself and learn. I always made a seating request in the beginning of the year. I asked that Gerard sit in the front of class so that he could concentrate on what was being taught and also stay away from any distraction in the back of the room.

Driving

Gerard started practicing driving through our neighborhood and in my mom's small hometown. He progressed to driving on the streets to the local grocery store which is only a half mile away.

Despite having ADHD and dyslexia, he is a really good driver. He always remembers to put on his seatbelt before he puts the car in drive. There's one small problem however, he likes to listen to his music at a volume that I would consider as a distraction. He tells me that he can concentrate, but of course as a mom I feel that the volume would hinder him from focusing on the roadway. We compromise and he has the volume at a low-medium level. I registered him to take the DriveSmart Drivers Education Course which consists of two weekend courses (30 classroom hours) 9-5 Saturday and Sunday. He will then have 6 hours of driving on the road with an instructor. He can complete those hours when he wants in any increment. This is a perfect way for him to learn everything about driving and the roads, hazards, and signs. Gerard received his license March 14, 1016. He was so excited. I allowed him to drive me home which was about 14 miles. He did fine even thought my heart was about to jump out of my chest. Since earning his license, he had caused considerable damage too my bumper by hitting the garage…oh my! My insurance company, pockets, and I am not ready for him to drive alone.

Medicine

Should I have placed Gerard on medicine? I had a visit with his pediatrician concerning his ADHD. His ADHD was not a problem for me and the teachers were not complaining in fourth grade. She suggested only if I was willing; that we try Strattera, which is a nonstimulant medication. I agreed to try it for three weeks and then we would visit her again as a follow-up. She suggested that we try it over the weekend so we could determine if he had any reaction to the medicine. We started him on the medicine on a Friday morning. The requirements of the medicine were to take with a meal. He ate before and after taking the medicine. The entire weekend he stayed nauseated. I could not continue this medicine, so I called his pediatrician on Mondaymorning. This medicine was available in 2003 in the United States; however, in 2005 the FDA warned of an increased risk of suicidal thinking in youth.

I am extremely happy that I did not continue the medicine. Gerard's pediatrician suggested we try a different drug since the first one had a negative effect. Vyvanse was the newly prescribed medicine. It is a central nervous system stimulant. It affects chemicals in the brain and nerves that contribute to hyperactivity and impulse control. I read really good reviews about vyvanse and was excited to have a test trial for Gerard. The first day went well, with no problems such as nausea or a headache. Two days after we tried vyvanse, he walked down our stairs and told me that his legs feel shaky. I learned thaVyvanse can cause rapid or irregular heartbeat, delirium, panic, psychosis, and heart failure. At that moment, I determined that I would not subject him to medicine that would alter his mood and physical form. I felt really sad for him at that moment because I told him the pill that he was taking was a vitamin. He trusted me and I lied to him.

I felt better knowing that I would not have to lie to him any more since he would not take any more medicine. I contacted his pediatrician to provide the details of the reaction to the pills. I told her that I felt more comfortable with him not being on any medicine and she agreed with me about the potential side effects. She told me it was my decision and she was proud that I was willing to work with him at home and school to help him succeed. My son's grandmother does not believe that conventional medicine helps at all times. She sent me Dhea, omega 6, and a multi-vitamin. He started the combination of vitamins in fourth grade, now he is in tenth grade and still using the same method to help with concentration and focus.

ADHD Coaching

After helping Gerard for sixteen years, I decided that it was time for me to provide assistance to other children and their parents. I had 'winged' the whole process of helping my son from birth to present time. I did what I thought was best for him and it just happened to work. He is now successful, happy, and learning new subjects in tenth grade at school, doing things at home and in the community. People with ADHD typically need help with setting goals and prioritizing, directing attention to the task at hand, creating and sticking to timelines and staying focused. Coaching helps them with time management, organizational skills and building self-esteem.

With encouragement and coaching, Gerard stays motivated. I have noticed his confidence and self-esteem has increased tremendously since I dedicated my time and effort to working with him. When I affirm his success in school, SAT/ACT studying, or home chores it increases his motivation to follow through on the learned systems that he knows are working. As an ADHD coach my plan is to help my son focus on understanding his needs as I teach him to set goals for changing old behavior patterns and creating new ones. For years I worked with my son to create an environment that was supportive so he could discover how to replace his negative thoughts, feelings and behaviors with positive patterns for success. He inevitably enjoyed the journey of learning more about himself and how ADHD plays a role in his life, which in turn can help him learn about how his ADHD brain works and become more effective at home, at school, and in extra-curricular activities. I taught Gerard to realize that ADHD was never going to go away. I taught him to learn the factors of his ADHD and to strategize to become successful.

I truly believe coaching accomplishes two things. It creates a pathway for learning and it helps those with ADHD understand their weaknesses and strengths so that they can capitalize. I have helped Gerard concentrate on his individual skills that will help balance his lifestyle. He prides himself on loving chaos. He considers chaos as clothes on the floor, bed unmade, or papers stashed in his backpack. Structure is one of the most difficult elements for him to follow. I make sure he lays out his clothes and his brother packs his backpack before school. I also make sure that he writes his schedule for the week in his planner. In order for him to move forward he will need to have structure in his daily life. The more success he has with structure, the more he will want to keep and follow a routine. As I mentioned, Gerard is not a fan of structure or time. I developed strength based strategies that would help him estimate time. I had him create a start and stop time for planning his daily activities. He set an alarm on his iPhone that would sound when it was time for him to finish planning. At times he found it difficult to plan properly as he was not focusing on the more in depth planning that was needed for him to manage his time. He finally decided to concentrate on his planning since it decreased the anxiety for the week.

When my son was in second grade I bought a timer with a buzzer that would signify when time was up on a task. I even use the timer when he takes a shower, since he is 16 now he manages to stay in the shower for 30 minutes or more. I had to cut shower time down, so I now have him shower for less than 10 minutes, which is more than enough time. Our mornings are sometimes crazy when I don't focus on time and I am late by a few minutes telling the boys that they have a few minutes before we leave. I try to give them at least 1 hour and 10 minutes to get up, get dressed, and eat breakfast. Every morning my son is late coming to the table. So this year, I set his timer 20 minutes before he should be at the table. Setting the timer has helped him stay on task and get to the table on time to have breakfast without added anxiety.

If your child is similar to my son, then they are able to "pull it off in the ninth hour". I am sure this action can be frustrating for parents, but by incorporating useful strategies your child will be able to devise methods to stay on track. Gerard and I have developed a 12 month calendar with pages that are easy to read and write in using the supplied colored markers. When there is a deadline for a project you could help your child establish and meet a minimal goal. Begin by defining the smallest possible goal that will accomplish something meaningful on the project or task. This task should be called the minimal goal and you and he should schedule a time to complete it. At the scheduled time, make sure he does only the minimal, even if it is watching a five minute video. This will allow him to approach a small part of the project without feeling overwhelmed.

As I have mentioned, Gerard is impulsive, a classic characteristic of ADHD. He does things before he thinks about intended actions, he leaps before he looks with nothing to guide him. He lacks impulse control and therefore speaks his mind even when no one asks. He blurts out things, interrupts people'sconversations and these actions may sometimes breeds resentment between him and many of his cohorts. I am happy he has friends who understand and love him regardless of his impulsivity. Strategically, I have worked with Gerard and clients to help them become aware of their impulsivity. I tell him that before he blurts out something, he should ask himself one question: "is this appropriate and are they talking to me?" I ask my clients and son to ask a close friend for feedback on their behavior. Feedback can be invaluable in helping to know how they come across. It helps them learn to better self-observe and avoid talking too much or too loudly. My son's best friend will tap my son's hand when he is talking too much in a group; this action has saved my son from standing out on multiple occasions.

When searching for papers from school Gerard has a difficult time finding it in his backpack because it is usually filled with papers from the previous four months. When we encounter this issue, I ask him why his backpack is so cluttered. He normally remarks that he became distracted in class and did not put the paper in the proper section of his binder. This lack of organizational skills has led to many nights of me helping him re-organize his binder with color coded dividers. One great advantage of having ADHD is the ability to have many solutions to one problem. For example, Gerard can see and pay attention to many things at once, while others focus on only one thing. Although it is beneficial to be distracted, there are on the other hand disadvantages too. Although it would appear that he is distracted, to me he lacked planning and prioritizing skills. He has a difficult time determining what the most important task to complete is, so he doesn't plan tocomplete the most important one.

To help Gerard when he becomes distracted, I have him visualize what he needs to do for the day. He has his planner that is located on the website. He sits down for a few minutes in the morning and reviews what events, homework, and projects are due for the day. It is now six months before the SAT and ACT and he is preparing to take the both in October. I am working with him to focus on this long term goal. He was under the understanding that he could start studying in August and take the test in October. I have him study his hardest subject for at least two months. There are 4 subjects on the test, so he will study and review each subject for two months. To rid any distractibility he studies in his room at his desk while his brother is in his room with no music, phone, or computer.

On the weekend he studies for at least 1 hour and during the weekday, he reviews for at least 10 minutes every afternoon. He is practicing track every afternoon for two hours every day and he has a meet every Saturday. I try not to overwhelm him during the week considering he has track practice and homework. I divided the task of studying into smaller, more manageable pieces. When he finishes a subject he will mark it check and move on to the next subject. This will give him a feeling of achievement and success while studying for the test which eludes a majority of students and causes them to freak out.

Chapter Six
Parent Advice

"What lies behind us and what lies before us are tiny matters compared to what lies within us." ~Ralph Waldo Emerson

Practicing forgiveness can be very difficult to do daily, but I have found that meditation in the morning helps me forgive anything that happened the previous day. I have also forgiven myself for saying things to Gerard when I was caught up in a moment of frustration. I also asked him if he would also forgive me for those things that I said and he has agreed on numerous occasions. I would never want to hurt his feelings because I know for sure at times he can't control his impulses. I admit that there have been situations with him that have left me angry and anxious and therefore physically provoked to call him a name that I should never have in life. I have forgiven myself, as should you if you are like me. Children with ADHD have the capacity to bring out the worst in parents, which frequently leaves parents feeling terribly guilty over their own actions. I feel that I am work under construction and I am built from foundation to infrastructure, now I am a strong and in the position to lead him where he needs to be in life.

I have always loved to work out and my endorphins thank me when I leave the gym because all of my worries and stress leave my mind and body. I have shared some things that I do to help me cope with my son's ADHD. I joined a social jogging club. We jog together 3 days during the week. As I mentioned I also work out on my own at the gym with my music blasting in my ears. I meditate for at least 3 minutes in the morning before anyone else wakes up. I like to take time in the morning to hear my own thoughts, my fears, and my ambitions for the day. Parents should take coach-approach with their kids, communicating more effectively to get better results. Rather than just managing difficult behaviors, parents should help their children thrive and become more independent.

Raising a child with ADHD can be a frustrating and overwhelming experience. Each and every one of us already has our struggles in life and these make parenting even a perfectly healthy child challenging. However we must realize that deep within us lies the ability to bring up that beautiful child and help him or her to achieve all of their potential. As a parent you have a very important role to play in controlling and reducing the symptoms and adverse effects of ADHD. Your child will face challenges everyday carrying out simple tasks that most people take for granted and will need you to smoothen the way for him. They will need guidance with channeling all that energy into positive areas of their lives that will enable them harness their innate skills and talents.

In a sense, you will need to micro-manage your child in order for them to get through the day. This means that they will need constant guidance and monitoring while you train them to acquire their own executive skills. When your child with ADHD annoys, ignores or embarrasses you, it is important for you to remember that they are not being willful or disobedient. They actually want to keep themselves tidy and organized or sit quietly like their fellow children and carry out the instructions you give them – but they are simply unable to do these things. Keeping this in mind will help you to empathize with your child and make it easier for you to respond to their symptoms with love and affirmation. Believe me, it is possible to raise a child with ADHD and still have a happy and stable home.

Your child's symptoms will not only impact you as the parent, but will also affect every member of your family. Their inability to process instructions will mean that they will not obey those instructions. When they get distracted and are disorganized it can delay other family members. Kids with ADHD are prone to beginning a task and then trailing off with another idea and this will leave someone else in the family with the task of cleaning up after them. They could speak and butt into conversations that do not concern them, often saying embarrassing or tactless things because they do not think before they speak. Getting a child with

ADHD to sit still and stop playing rough games that will endanger their lives is difficult, as is trying to put them to bed at night. As a parent you will face challenges interacting with them too because it can be physically exhausting trying to meet the demands of a child with ADHD. Having to monitor them constantly to make sure that they are not unconsciously putting themselves in harm's way will also take its toll on your psyche. It will be frustrating when your child does not 'listen' to you. A build up of this frustration can lead to anger which will in turn lead to guilt about being angry at your own child. Their condition will also affect their siblings who will feel that they are getting less attention than the child with ADHD whilst having to shoulder some of the responsibility of taking care of the child.

It has been a long journey from my child's diagnosis to this place and I can tell you that I have learned a lot and developed as a person through all of it. My advice to parents is that you first and foremost ensure that you stay healthy and positive yourself because you cannot help your child if you do not have a positive attitude and mindset. Structure is very useful and will go a long way in ensuring that things get done and no part of your life or that of any member of your family is neglected. Ensure that you communicate clearly and simply to the child with ADHD so that he can understand your instructions. If you do these three things, I can assure you that you will successfully raise your child and live a full life while you're at it. I asked Gerard if he wanted to write a paragraph in the book to encourage boys. He said, "Mom I have only a few words for them. Tell them to have fun." I said, "but you struggled when you were young". He said, yeah I struggled when I was young, but I had fun on the playground. So tell your boys to have fun!

Made in the USA
Monee, IL
24 June 2021

72227738R10028